COMPLETE GUIDE TO UNDERSTANDING RHINOPLASTY

Essential Information, Recovery Tips, Best Practices For Nose Surgery, Cosmetic Enhancements, And Breathing Improvements

KLEIN HOYLE

Disclaimer

The content in this book is based on the author's expertise and comprehension of the topic. The author has no affiliation or link with any corporation, business, or person. This book is meant to give general information and educational material only, and it should not be interpreted as professional medical advice. Always seek the advice of a skilled healthcare expert if you have any queries about medical issues or treatments. The author and publisher expressly disclaim any responsibility resulting directly or indirectly from the use or use of the information included in this book.

Table of Contents

ABOUT THIS BOOK

The "Complete Guide to Understanding Rhinoplasty" is an invaluable resource for anybody considering or having rhinoplasty, providing a thorough examination of every aspect of this transforming treatment. At its heart, this book offers a fundamental knowledge of rhinoplasty, diving into its historical origins and explaining how it evolved into the complex surgical discipline that it is today. It emphasizes the critical function of informed consultation, highlighting the need for good communication between patient and surgeon in defining expectations and attaining optimum outcomes.

A comprehensive grasp of nasal anatomy is essential for navigating the complexities of rhinoplasty, and this tutorial pays special emphasis to this element. Readers will learn about the intricate interaction of cartilage and bone that defines nose anatomy, as well as the physiological mechanics that underpin nasal function. Furthermore, it tackles typical nasal disorders and their causes, allowing people to understand the underlying reasons for their desire for surgical intervention.

Preparing for rhinoplasty is a complicated task, and Chapter 3 carefully guides readers through the process. This section covers everything from choosing a competent surgeon to physically and emotionally preparing for the surgery, ensuring that people go into their surgeries well-prepared and knowledgeable. Furthermore, it clarifies the numerous kinds of rhinoplasty treatments, distinguishing between open and closed approaches, main and revision surgeries, and functional and cosmetic improvements. Ethnic issues are also carefully considered, taking into account the many anatomical peculiarities that exist among different groups.

Navigating the surgical procedure may be difficult, but Chapter 5 provides a thorough guide, from anesthetic choices to post-operative care. This book enables people to navigate their recovery path with confidence and resilience by explaining possible difficulties and management options. Chapter 6 delves more into the postoperative experience, explaining reasonable expectations, comprehending the healing process, and dealing with transient side effects including swelling and bruising.

Undoubtedly, rhinoplasty, like any surgical treatment, has inherent risks and consequences, and Chapter 7 provides readers with the information they need to limit these risks as well as detect and manage difficulties that may emerge. Furthermore, the need for meticulous postoperative care and follow-up sessions is emphasized, assuring excellent results and long-term pleasure.

Beyond the immediate postoperative period, Chapter 9 dives into the psychological and emotional elements of life after rhinoplasty, leading patients through the process of adapting to their new look and integrating their results into their everyday lives. Finally, it looks at alternatives to rhinoplasty, including information on non-surgical improvements and lifestyle changes for nasal health and beauty.

In conclusion, the "Complete Guide to Understanding Rhinoplasty" goes beyond the typical confines of a medical textbook, functioning as a beacon of information, empowerment, and direction for anyone starting their rhinoplasty adventure. Its comprehensive approach not only clarifies the surgical procedure but also encourages a better knowledge of the tremendous effects rhinoplasty may have on both physical appearance and psychological well-being.

CHAPTER 1

Introduction To Rhinoplasty

What Is Rhinoplasty?

Rhinoplasty, sometimes known as a "nose job," is a surgical operation that involves changing the shape, size, or proportions of the nose to enhance its look or function. It is one of the most common cosmetic operations in the world, with people seeking it for a variety of reasons, including improving face harmony, fixing breathing issues, and treating abnormalities caused by accidents or congenital disorders.

A Brief History Of Rhinoplasty

Rhinoplasty dates back thousands of years. Ancient civilizations, such as the Egyptians and Romans, used basic types of nose reconstruction surgery to mend injuries acquired in war or punishment.

However, contemporary rhinoplasty as we know it today started to emerge in the late nineteenth century, when pioneering surgeons devised more advanced procedures for nasal restoration.

Rhinoplasty procedures advanced in the early twentieth century, with surgeons experimenting with new ways to improve cosmetic outcomes. Rhinoplasty grew safer and more accessible to a wider variety of patients as anesthetic and surgical equipment improved. Rhinoplasty is now a highly developed surgical treatment that provides patients with both cosmetic and functional benefits while posing a low risk.

The Importance Of Proper Consultation

Before getting rhinoplasty, it is essential to have a comprehensive consultation with an experienced plastic surgeon. During this appointment, the surgeon will assess your nasal anatomy, talk about your objectives and expectations, and go over the possible risks and advantages of the treatment. This first visit also allows you to ask questions, voice your worries, and have a better knowledge of what to anticipate before, during, and after surgery.

A comprehensive consultation lays the groundwork for a successful rhinoplasty procedure. It helps the surgeon to personalize the treatment to your specific requirements and ensures that you have reasonable expectations for the outcome. Furthermore, the consultation allows you to evaluate the surgeon's credentials, expertise, and approach to rhinoplasty, making you feel more confident and educated as you proceed with the choice to have surgery.

Understanding Different Types Of Rhinoplasty

Rhinoplasty is not a one-size-fits-all treatment; rather, it includes a variety of procedures aimed at addressing particular cosmetic or functional issues. Some popular forms of rhinoplasty are:

1. Cosmetic Rhinoplasty: This form of rhinoplasty is intended merely to improve the look of the nose. It might include contouring the nasal tip, lowering or increasing the size of the nose, correcting asymmetry, or refining the nasal bridge.

2. Functional Rhinoplasty: This procedure seeks to enhance nasal function by treating concerns such as breathing difficulty, nasal congestion, or nasal valve collapse. This might include correcting a deviated septum, restoring nasal valve collapse, or lowering turbinate size to optimize airflow.

3. Revision Rhinoplasty, also known as secondary rhinoplasty, is a treatment used to rectify problems or disappointing outcomes from a prior rhinoplasty surgery. Addressing scar tissue, structural problems, and cosmetic issues that were not addressed during the first surgery demands a high degree of skill and knowledge.

4. Ethnic Rhinoplasty: Ethnic rhinoplasty is designed to address the specific anatomical characteristics and cultural preferences of people from various ethnic backgrounds. It seeks to improve the nose while keeping ethnic character and avoiding excessive Westernization.

Understanding the various forms of rhinoplasty allows patients to successfully communicate their objectives and expectations throughout the consultation process. By discussing your issues and intended objectives with your surgeon, you may work together to create a personalized treatment plan that provides natural-looking results while also meeting your practical and cosmetic demands.

CHAPTER 2

Anatomy Of The Nose

Understanding Nasal Structure

The human nose is a complicated structure made up of many components such as bone, cartilage, skin, and mucous membrane. Its form and size vary widely across people, adding to the distinctiveness of facial characteristics. The nasal anatomy is roughly separated into exterior and interior components.

Externally, the nose is made up of nasal bones (which create the bridge) and cartilage (which forms the tip and sides). The skin that covers these tissues dictates how the nose appears. The nasal cavity is a hollow area split into two channels by the nasal septum, which is composed of cartilage and bone.

The Function Of Cartilage And Bone In Nasal Shape

Cartilage and bone are important factors in shaping the form and structure of the nose. The nasal bones support the nasal bridge and help to determine its height and breadth. In contrast, cartilage shapes the nasal tip and sides, allowing for flexibility and movement.

The lower lateral cartilages, also known as alar cartilages, support the nasal tip and sides. During rhinoplasty, these cartilages may be moved around to change the shape and appearance of the nose. Surgeons may sculpt, trim, or relocate the cartilage to obtain the desired cosmetic results.

Understanding the interaction between cartilage and bone is critical for both patients and surgeons throughout the rhinoplasty procedure. By carefully modifying these tissues, surgeons may improve the look of the nose while preserving its function and structural integrity.

How Nasal Passages Work

The nasal passages perform various critical activities, such as humidifying, warming, and filtering the air we breathe. When we breathe in, air enters the nostrils and travels into the nasal cavity, where it is conditioned before reaching the lungs. This procedure protects the respiratory system from hazardous particles and germs.

The nasal septum splits the nasal cavity into two passageways, facilitating effective ventilation while preventing air from escaping via the mouth. Turbinates are mucous membrane-covered structures within the nasal cavity that assist control of airflow and improve air conditioning.

Understanding the structure and function of the nasal passageways is critical for diagnosing nasal problems and identifying the best treatment option, including rhinoplasty. To ensure that patients have the best possible results, surgeons must evaluate how changes to the nasal anatomy may influence airflow and breathing.

Common Nasal Issues And Causes

Nasal difficulties may be caused by a variety of circumstances, including congenital anomalies, severe traumas, and aging. Common nasal issues include a deviated septum, nasal congestion, deformities, and breathing difficulty.

A deviated septum develops when the nasal septum is crooked or misplaced, causing airflow blockage and breathing difficulties. Traumatic injuries, such as nose fractures, may result in anatomical abnormalities and functional limitations.

Age-related changes, such as cartilage loss and skin elasticity, may affect the look and function of the nose over time. These modifications may cause nasal tip drooping, nasal hump development, and breathing difficulty.

Understanding the origins of nose problems is critical for choosing the best treatment plan, including if rhinoplasty is required. Rhinoplasty, which addresses both cosmetic problems and functional limitations, may dramatically enhance patients' quality of life and self-esteem.

CHAPTER 3

Preparation For Rhinoplasty

Finding The Right Surgeon

Choosing the appropriate physician for your rhinoplasty treatment is critical to getting the results you want. Start by looking for certified and experienced surgeons in your region. Search for board-certified plastic surgeons or otolaryngologists who specialize in face plastic surgery.

When examining possible surgeons, look at their qualifications, expertise, and before-and-after images of former patients. Reading reviews and testimonials may also provide details about the surgeon's bedside manner and patient satisfaction.

It is critical to plan meetings with many surgeons to discuss your objectives, concerns, and expectations for the treatment.

During these discussions, pay attention to how the surgeon listens to your concerns and outlines their strategy for reaching your desired result.

The Consultation And Evaluation Process

The consultation and assessment procedure is an important step in preparing for rhinoplasty. This is where you may fully discuss your aims and expectations with your surgeon.

During the consultation, your surgeon will assess your nose structure, skin thickness, and overall face harmony. They will also go over the surgical approaches that may be appropriate for your specific condition and offer a realistic estimate of the outcomes you might anticipate.

Prepare to ask questions at the appointment to ensure that you fully understand the surgery, recovery process, and any risks and consequences. It is critical to have open and honest communication with your surgeon to ensure that you are both on the same page about your objectives and expectations.

Preoperative Instructions And Precautions

Before having a rhinoplasty, your surgeon will give you certain pre-operative instructions to follow. These guidelines may include food restrictions, medication adjustments, and lifestyle changes designed to improve your health and reduce the chance of problems.

Common pre-operative recommendations may include quitting smoking and drinking alcohol, avoiding certain drugs that increase the risk of bleeding, and making arrangements for transportation to and from the surgical facility.

Follow your surgeon's instructions closely to ensure you're in the best possible shape for surgery. Failure to follow pre-operative instructions may cause surgical delays or raise the risk of problems during and after the treatment.

Mental And Emotional Preparations For Surgery

Preparing psychologically and emotionally for rhinoplasty is as crucial as physical preparation. Understandably, having surgery may cause worry, dread, and uncertainty.

It is reasonable to be concerned about the result of the treatment and how it may affect your look. Take time to discuss any thoughts or anxiety you may have with your surgeon or a mental health expert.

Visualize your desired result and remember why you opted to get rhinoplasty in the first place. Surround yourself with friends and family who will encourage and reassure you during the process.

Relaxation practices such as deep breathing, meditation, or yoga may help manage tension and produce a feeling of calm in the run-up to surgery. To guarantee a successful rhinoplasty procedure, trust your surgeon's competence and the thorough preparation you've done.

CHAPTER 4

Types Of Rhinoplasty Procedures

Open Vs. Closed Rhinoplasty

Understanding the approach

When it comes to rhinoplasty treatments, one of the most important distinguishing factors is whether surgeons utilize open or closed techniques. These phrases allude to how the surgeon gets to the nasal structures during surgery.

Open Rhinoplasty: A Clearer View.

An open rhinoplasty involves the surgeon making an incision across the columella, a band of tissue that separates the nostrils. This enables the surgeon to peel the skin away from the underlying nasal tissues, offering a clear view of the anatomy. With such good sight, the surgeon may precisely remodel the nose, addressing both cosmetic and functional issues with accuracy.

Closed Rhinoplasty with Concealed Incisions

In contrast, a closed rhinoplasty involves making incisions fully within the nostrils. This method is less invasive since it does not need an exterior incision in the columella. While it reduces direct exposure of nasal components, qualified surgeons may still conduct intricate nose remodeling via the nostril apertures.

Choosing the Right Approach

The choice between open and closed rhinoplasty is often determined by the precise aims of the operation as well as the surgeon's experience. Open rhinoplasty may be used for more difficult situations requiring perfect visualization, although closed rhinoplasty may serve for minor cosmetic modifications.

Primary Versus Revision Rhinoplasty

Starting Fresh vs. Corrective Surgery

Rhinoplasty is divided into two forms depending on the aim of the procedure: primary and revision rhinoplasty.

Primary Rhinoplasty: Making the Initial Change.

Primary rhinoplasty is the initial nasal surgery done on a patient. Whether the objective is to improve nasal function or enhance the look of the nose, primary rhinoplasty enables surgeons to work with the natural nasal architecture without making any previous changes. It's an opportunity to shape the nose according to the patient's preferences while remaining in harmony with their facial characteristics.

Revision Rhinoplasty: Correcting Previous Work.

In contrast, revision rhinoplasty is done to resolve issues or complications from prior nasal surgery.

It necessitates a greater degree of competence owing to the changed nasal structure and scar tissue caused by the previous treatment. Surgeons doing revision rhinoplasty must manage existing modifications while attempting to accomplish the patient's desired objective of restoring both form and function.

Complexities and Considerations

Revision rhinoplasty may be more difficult than original rhinoplasty owing to the unpredictable nature of scar tissue and the risk of impaired nasal structure. Patients needing revision surgery should choose a surgeon with expertise in doing difficult nasal revisions to achieve the best possible outcomes.

Functional Vs. Aesthetic Rhinoplasty

Balancing Form and Function

Rhinoplasty is not just for improving the look of the nose; it may also address functional concerns that impair breathing and general nasal function. Understanding the difference between functional and cosmetic rhinoplasty is critical for people contemplating nose surgery.

Aesthetic Rhinoplasty: Enhancing Appearance.

Aesthetic rhinoplasty aims to improve the visual appearance of the nose. The objective is to achieve a more harmonic and balanced face profile, whether that means decreasing a pronounced dorsal hump, refining the nasal tip, or addressing asymmetry. To produce natural-looking results, surgeons doing aesthetic rhinoplasty must take into account the patient's face dimensions, skin thickness, and aesthetic preferences.

Functional Rhinoplasty Improves Nasal Function

Functional rhinoplasty corrects anatomical abnormalities in the nose that prevent appropriate breathing or nasal airflow.

This might include correcting a deviated septum, decreasing nasal turbinates, or restoring nasal valve collapse. Functional rhinoplasty may also have cosmetic advantages since it restores appropriate nasal function, which typically results in a more balanced nasal look.

Combining Aesthetic and Functional Goals

In many situations, rhinoplasty surgeries combine cosmetic and functional changes. Surgeons must strike a delicate balance between the patient's cosmetic goals and the necessity to preserve or enhance nasal function. This complete approach guarantees that patients not only accomplish their cosmetic goals but also have better breathing and nasal health.

Ethnic Rhinoplasty Considerations

Respecting Cultural Diversity

Ethnic rhinoplasty understands that nasal anatomy differs between nationalities and civilizations. While the fundamental principles of nose surgery remain unchanged, doctors who perform ethnic rhinoplasty must understand and respect each ethnic group's distinct aesthetic standards and physical traits.

Cultural Diversity in Nasal Anatomy

Ethnic rhinoplasty includes operations designed for people of African, Asian, Hispanic, Middle Eastern, and other ethnic origins. These groups may have unique nasal characteristics, such as broader nasal bases, thicker skin, or poorer nasal cartilage support. Surgeons who specialize in ethnic rhinoplasty understand how to address these variances while keeping the patient's cultural identity and face harmony.

Customized Treatment Plans

Ethnic rhinoplasty necessitates a tailored approach that takes into account the patient's ethnic origin, face dimensions, and aesthetic preferences. Surgeons may use specialized procedures, such as cartilage grafting or tip refining, to generate natural-looking outcomes that highlight the patient's distinctive attractiveness while preserving their cultural background.

Cultural Sensitivity and Communication

Patients having ethnic rhinoplasty should be assured that their surgeon knows and respects their cultural heritage. Clear communication between the patient and surgeon is critical to ensuring that the surgery plan meets the patient's cosmetic objectives while respecting their ethnic identity. Surgeons may create attractive and meaningful outcomes in ethnic rhinoplasty surgeries by putting cultural awareness and tailored care first.

CHAPTER 5

The Rhinoplasty Surgery Process

Anesthesia Options And Risks

Before getting into the complexities of rhinoplasty surgery, it's critical to understand the anesthetic alternatives and the dangers involved. Anesthesia is essential for maintaining the patient's comfort and safety during the treatment. There are two main forms of anesthesia used in rhinoplasty: local anesthesia with sedation and general anesthesia.

Local anesthesia with sedation entails numbing the surgical region while keeping the patient comfortable and sleepy with sedatives delivered intravenously. This approach permits patients to stay awake during the surgery, although in a profoundly relaxed condition.

It is often recommended for less sophisticated rhinoplasty procedures and has a faster recovery period than general anesthesia.

General anesthesia, on the other hand, causes the patient to become entirely asleep and unresponsive throughout the operation. This option is sometimes used for more complex rhinoplasty treatments or for individuals who are frightened or uncomfortable with the prospect of being awake throughout surgery. However, it has a greater risk of complications, including allergic responses, respiratory difficulties, and postoperative nausea and vomiting.

Each anesthetic approach has unique risks and advantages that should be extensively reviewed with the surgeon during pre-operative consultations. The patient's medical history, the intricacy of the surgery, and personal preferences will all impact the kind of anesthetic used. Patients should also report any allergies, drugs, or pre-existing diseases to ensure a safe anesthetic experience.

A Step-By-Step Overview Of The Surgical Procedure

Rhinoplasty surgery, sometimes known as a nose job, is a sophisticated and highly customized treatment that reshapes the nose to enhance its look and function. While the details of the operation may differ based on the patient's anatomy and intended goal, a broad step-by-step outline might help explain the procedure.

1. **Preparation:** Before the procedure, the patient is prepared and placed on the operating table. Anesthesia is used to ensure the patient's comfort throughout the surgery.

2. **Incisions:** Depending on the surgical strategy selected (open or closed rhinoplasty), the surgeon makes discrete incisions within the nostrils (closed rhinoplasty) or across the columella (open). These incisions provide access to the underlying structures of the nose.

3. Reshaping: After gaining access to the nasal structures, the surgeon meticulously reshapes the bone, cartilage, and soft tissue to produce the desired cosmetic result. Osteotomies (bone cutting), cartilage grafting, and tip refining are used to shape the nose based on the patient's preferences.

4. Closure: After the reshaping is completed, the wounds are precisely closed with sutures. In closed rhinoplasty, the incisions are concealed inside the nostrils, but in open rhinoplasty, the little exterior incision is discreetly positioned along the columella.

5. Postoperative Care: Following surgery, the patient is constantly observed in the recovery room to facilitate a seamless transition from anesthesia. Pain relievers and antibiotics may be provided to alleviate pain and prevent infection. Patients get extensive postoperative advice to help them recuperate properly and avoid problems.

Possible Complications And How They Are Managed

While rhinoplasty is typically safe and successful, it can have certain risks and problems, as with any surgical surgery. Understanding these risks and how they are handled is critical for making sound decisions and achieving optimum results.

Possible Complications Of Rhinoplasty Include:

• Prompt action is necessary to reduce excessive bleeding during or after surgery and avoid problems like hematoma development.

• Infections may still arise after surgery, even with strict sterile procedures. Prompt diagnosis and antibiotic treatment are critical for preventing infection spread and reducing tissue damage.

• Nasal blockage might continue or worsen following surgery due to edema, scarring, or poor healing.

This may impair breathing and need extra treatments such as revision surgery or steroid injections.

• Minor asymmetries or abnormalities may develop during rhinoplasty, despite the goal of achieving perfect symmetry and smooth outlines. These may often be treated with revision surgery or nonsurgical methods like injectable fillers.

Managing these problems requires a joint effort between the surgeon and the patient, as well as careful monitoring and quick treatments when necessary. Patients should strictly adhere to all postoperative instructions and attend all follow-up consultations to ensure that any concerns are handled as soon as possible.

Postoperative Care And Recovery Timeline

The effectiveness of rhinoplasty surgery is determined not only by surgical expertise but also by attentive postoperative care and adherence to the specified recovery timeframe. Proper recovery care is essential for lowering pain, and swelling, and supporting optimum healing.

During the first days after surgery, patients might expect:

• Swelling and bruising around the nose and eyes are normal after rhinoplasty, peaking within 48 hours and then receding over weeks.

• Nasal packing or splints may be used to support newly remodeled structures and reduce edema. These are often removed during the first week after surgery.

• Restricted Activities: Patients should avoid intense activities, leaning over, and carrying heavy things during early recovery to minimize problems including bleeding or disturbance of healing wounds.

As the initial swelling subsides, patients will see incremental improvements in the look and function of their noses. However, complete recovery and ultimate outcomes may take several months to a year as residual swelling diminishes and the tissues adjust to their new form.

Patients should communicate openly with their surgeon throughout the healing process, mentioning any concerns or unexpected symptoms as soon as possible. Following all postoperative instructions, attending regular follow-up visits, and being patient are critical to getting the greatest potential results following rhinoplasty surgery.

CHAPTER 6

Rhinoplasty Results And Expectations

Reasonable Predictions For The Outcomes Of Rhinoplasty

Setting reasonable expectations is critical for anybody contemplating rhinoplasty. surgery is important to note that, although rhinoplasty might improve your look and confidence, surgery does not guarantee perfection. Communicating candidly with your surgeon about your objectives and knowing what is attainable for your specific anatomy is critical.

During your appointment, your surgeon will go over the possible results of rhinoplasty depending on your issues and desired improvements. They will also evaluate your nose anatomy and skin thickness to determine the feasibility of reaching your objectives. Remember that everyone's outcomes will differ, and what is doable for one person may be impossible for another.

It's critical to recognize the limits of rhinoplasty and approach the treatment with reasonable expectations. While rhinoplasty may help with cosmetic and practical difficulties, it may not entirely improve your look or remove all flaws. Understanding this ahead may assist in avoiding disappointment and achieving a more fulfilling end.

Understanding The Healing Process

After rhinoplasty, the healing period is critical since it dictates the ultimate result of the treatment. Understanding what to anticipate throughout the healing process might assist in reducing anxiety and promote a smoother recovery.

Swelling, bruising, and pain around the nose and eyes are likely to occur immediately after surgery. Your surgeon will give you special post-operative advice to assist control your symptoms and encourage recovery. To avoid issues and get the best outcomes, please follow these directions.

Swelling will progressively reduce in the weeks after surgery, and you will start to notice the benefits of your rhinoplasty. However, it is important to remember that the ultimate result may not be visible for many months after surgery, since residual edema takes time to decrease completely.

It is common for your look to fluctuate throughout the healing process as edema reduces and tissues settle. It's important to be patient and let your body recover naturally. Avoiding rigorous activities and according to your surgeon's suggestions will assist in ensuring a faster recovery and better long-term outcomes.

Long-Term Results And Possible Changes Over Time

While rhinoplasty may yield long-term improvements, it's important to remember that your nose may continue to change over time. Aging, gravity, and weight fluctuations may all affect the look of your nose in the years after surgery.

Understanding the various changes that may occur over time will help you maintain reasonable expectations and prepare for future modifications as needed. While some people may obtain permanent results with rhinoplasty, others may need further touch-up surgeries to maintain their ideal look.

Regular follow-up meetings with your surgeon may help you track your progress and manage any issues that occur over time. By being proactive and communicating openly with your surgeon, you may ensure that your rhinoplasty results satisfy your long-term objectives.

Dealing With Temporary Swelling And Bruising

Rhinoplasty often causes swelling and bruising, which are usually transient. While these symptoms may be troubling at first, it is important to recognize that they are a typical component of the healing process and will progressively improve with time.

Your surgeon may prescribe a variety of measures to assist minimize swelling and bruising, including using cold compresses, elevating your head, and avoiding drugs that might cause bleeding or edema. Following these guidelines may reduce pain and encourage speedier recovery.

It's important to be patient throughout the healing process and let your body heal at its speed. While swelling and bruising may be evident at first, they will eventually subside, exposing the ultimate results of your rhinoplasty.

Meanwhile, concentrating on self-care and according to your surgeon's recommendations will help you recover more quickly and with a better result.

CHAPTER 7
Risks And Complications

Potential Risks Associated With Rhinoplasty

Rhinoplasty, like any other surgical surgery, has inherent risks and problems. Understanding the dangers is critical for anybody contemplating rhinoplasty.

Infection is a frequent concern, and it may happen despite the surgeon's best efforts to keep the setting clean. Infections may cause issues such as delayed healing and tissue damage. Another danger is bleeding, which may occur during or after the surgery. While some bleeding is normal, excessive bleeding may need extra medical treatment.

There is also a risk of anesthesia-related adverse events, including nausea, vomiting, and allergic responses. Anesthesia-related problems are uncommon but may occur, especially in those who have pre-existing medical disorders.

Other possible concerns include asymmetry or abnormalities in the nasal form, unhappiness with the cosmetic result, and difficulty breathing through the nose owing to structural alterations. These hazards differ according to the patient's anatomy, the procedure's intricacy, and the surgeon's ability and expertise.

How To Minimize Risks Before Surgery

Before undergoing rhinoplasty surgery, many precautions may be performed to reduce the dangers involved.

First and foremost, choose a board-certified plastic surgeon with substantial expertise in rhinoplasty. Researching possible doctors, reading patient reviews, and arranging appointments to discuss the treatment will help you choose a knowledgeable and competent physician.

Additionally, it is critical that you follow your surgeon's pre-operative instructions. This may involve refraining from taking drugs or supplements that raise the risk of bleeding, such as aspirin or ibuprofen. It is also critical that you inform your surgeon about any pre-existing medical issues or allergies since they might impact the surgical procedure and increase your risk of complications.

Maintaining a healthy lifestyle before surgery may also assist reduce risks. This includes eating a well-balanced diet, keeping hydrated, and quitting smoking, since smoking may slow recovery and raise the risk of problems.

Recognizing And Managing Complications After Surgery

Despite precautions, difficulties may still occur after rhinoplasty. It is critical to recognize the signals of possible problems and seek immediate medical assistance if they arise.

Excessive bleeding, intense pain or swelling, fever, and infection symptoms like as redness or discharge from the incision site are all common markers of problems. If you encounter any of these symptoms, you should call your surgeon immediately.

In certain circumstances, difficulties may need extra medical treatment, such as medications for an infection or surgical revision to correct asymmetry or other concerns. However, with good treatment, most issues may be successfully addressed without long-term repercussions.

The Significance Of Confirmation Meetings

Follow-up meetings with your surgeon are necessary to monitor your recovery and handle any concerns or issues that may occur. During these meetings, your surgeon may examine your progress, remove any packing or splints, and make any required changes to your treatment plan.

During follow-up meetings, your surgeon may also advise you on post-operative care, such as correct wound care procedures and when it is safe to resume regular activities. Furthermore, these sessions allow you to discuss your cosmetic objectives and verify that you are pleased with the outcome of your rhinoplasty.

Overall, following your surgeon's advice and attending all planned follow-up visits is critical to getting the greatest results from your rhinoplasty treatment. By being watchful and proactive throughout your recuperation, you may reduce the chance of problems while still enjoying the advantages of your newly improved nasal look.

CHAPTER 8
Post-Operative Care And Recovery

Immediate Postoperative Care Instructions

To guarantee a smooth recovery following rhinoplasty surgery, follow precise guidelines right away. When you wake up from anesthesia, you'll most likely be in a recovery room where medical professionals will monitor your status. You may feel groggy, nauseated, or uncomfortable at first. It's normal, and medical staff will help you manage these symptoms. You will also be given post-operative instructions, such as how to care for your nose, which medicines to take, and when to check up with your surgeon.

To decrease swelling and encourage appropriate healing, keep your head up at all times, even while sleeping.

This may be accomplished by utilizing many pillows to support oneself or by sleeping in a chair. It is also critical to avoid vigorous activity, such as bending over or carrying heavy things, during the early recuperation period.

Your surgeon would most likely advise you to refrain from blowing your nose for some time to avoid disrupting the healing process. Instead, gently smelling or cleaning the nose with a tissue is advised. Nasal congestion and moderate bleeding are normal in the first few days after surgery, and your surgeon may prescribe nasal sprays or saline solutions to help relieve these symptoms.

It's also important to keep hydrated and eat a healthy diet to help your body recuperate. Avoiding drinking and smoking is critical at this time since they may slow recovery and raise the chance of problems. Adhering to these post-operative care guidelines will help you heal faster and get the best outcomes from your rhinoplasty treatment.

Managing Discomfort And Pain

While discomfort and suffering are unavoidable after rhinoplasty surgery, there are numerous ways to properly manage these symptoms. Your surgeon will most likely prescribe pain relievers to assist lessen any discomfort you may feel. It is critical to take these drugs as prescribed and not wait until the pain gets severe before taking them.

In addition to pain relievers, using cold compresses on swollen parts of your face may be beneficial. Cold packs or bags of frozen peas wrapped in a towel may be gently placed on the cheeks and around the eyes to relieve swelling and numbness. To avoid frostbite or skin injury, ice should not be applied directly to the skin.

Relaxation methods such as deep breathing exercises or meditation may also assist with pain and discomfort. These tactics not only induce relaxation but also serve to divert you from any pain you may be feeling. Staying well-rested and avoiding intense activities might also help to reduce pain and discomfort throughout the healing process.

If you continue to have severe or prolonged pain after following these techniques, call your surgeon right away, since this might suggest a problem that needs urgent treatment. Open communication with your surgical team during the healing period is critical to ensuring a smooth and successful rhinoplasty surgery.

How To Care For Incisions And Dressings

Proper care of your wounds and dressings is critical for promoting healing and lowering the risk of infection after rhinoplasty surgery. Your surgeon will give you precise advice on how to care for your wounds and when to change dressings. you get the best outcomes from your operation, be sure you carefully follow these recommendations.

Steri-strips or thin bandages may be used to cover your wounds immediately after surgery. It is critical to keep these dressings clean and dry to avoid infection. Your surgeon may advise you to avoid getting the dressings wet in the shower and to carefully pat them dry if they do get moist.

As the healing process develops, your surgeon may remove the dressings or show you how to do it at home. It is critical to follow their instructions precisely to prevent disturbing the healing process or injuring the incisions. After the bandages are removed, your surgeon may suggest putting antibiotic ointment or moisturizer on the incision areas to aid healing and decrease scarring.

It's also important to avoid exposing your incisions to direct sunlight throughout the healing phase, since UV radiation may cause discoloration and slow recovery. If you must be in the sun, use sunscreen with a high SPF to protect your skin and incisions from harm.

If you see any indications of infection, such as increased redness, swelling, or discharge from the incision sites, call your surgeon right once. Infections must be treated promptly to avoid problems and guarantee a successful rhinoplasty surgery.

Slowly Get Back To Your Regular Activities

While it is natural to want to return to regular activities as soon as possible following rhinoplasty surgery, it is critical to do so gradually to minimize problems and encourage good recovery. Your surgeon will advise you on when it is safe to resume certain activities depending on your specific healing status.

It is critical to relax and avoid vigorous activities that may cause swelling or tension on the surgical site in the days after surgery. Light walking is usually suggested to improve circulation and prevent blood clots, but activities that require bending over or carrying heavy things should be avoided.

As the swelling and bruises decrease, you may gradually resume more typical tasks, such as moderate housework or office work. However, you must listen to your body and avoid pushing yourself too hard too quickly. If you feel any pain or exhaustion, take a pause and relax.

Most patients may return to work or school after 1-2 weeks of rhinoplasty surgery, depending on their career and personal healing status. However, for many weeks after surgery, avoid any activity that might raise the risk of nose damage, such as contact sports or hard lifting.

Finally, the timing for returning to regular activities will differ for each patient, so it is critical to attentively follow your surgeon's instructions to ensure a smooth and complete recovery following rhinoplasty surgery. Patience and attention throughout the recuperation period will result in better outcomes and a more pleasant end to your treatment.

CHAPTER 9

Life After Rhinoplasty

Psychological And Emotional Aspects Of Life After Rhinoplasty

Rhinoplasty involves both a physical and emotional makeover. It's typical to have a variety of emotions following surgery. Initially, you may be delighted about the changes to your appearance, but you may also feel nervous or even melancholy as you adjust to the new look. Understanding these feelings and allowing yourself time to process them is critical.

One frequent post-surgery sensation is a sense of vulnerability. Your nose is a prominent aspect of your face, therefore any changes to it may have an impact on your self-esteem and confidence. It's crucial to remember that the choice to have rhinoplasty was made for personal reasons, and the ultimate goal is to feel comfortable in your skin.

Friends, family, and your healthcare team can all help you get through this difficult time. Surround yourself with good influences and individuals that inspire you. Talking freely about your emotions might also assist in reducing any worries or anxieties you may have.

Patience is essential during the rehabilitation process. Your ultimate results may not be noticeable right away, and swelling and bruising are usual in the weeks that follow surgery. Be kind to yourself, and let your body recover at its rate. Remember that the route to your ideal look is slow.

Adjusting To Your New Appearance

Getting used to your new look after rhinoplasty may be both exhilarating and stressful. You may notice slight alterations in your facial characteristics that will take some adjusting to.

It is critical to have reasonable expectations for the result of the operation and to recognize that small flaws are common and may improve with time.

As you become used to your new nose, you may start experimenting with various haircuts, cosmetic methods, and clothing trends to complement your improved features. Take advantage of this chance to discover your style and express yourself in new ways.

It is very usual for people to notice and compliment you on your new look after rhinoplasty. While this is nice, keep in mind that your view is the most important. Concentrate on how you feel about your new appearance rather than seeking approval from others.

If you are dissatisfied with the outcomes of your rhinoplasty, do not hesitate to discuss it honestly with your surgeon. They may advise you on various revision surgeries or non-surgical treatments to address your concerns.

Maintenance And Follow-Up Care

Following rhinoplasty, thorough maintenance, and follow-up care are critical for achieving the best results and avoiding problems. Your surgeon will give you particular post-operative instructions, such as how to clean and protect your nose, as well as any drugs or therapies that will help with the healing process.

It is important to attend all planned follow-up sessions with your surgeon to track your progress and handle any issues that may emerge. During these sessions, your surgeon will evaluate the healing of your nose and advise you on when it is safe to resume typical activities, such as exercising and wearing glasses.

In addition according to your surgeon's instructions, you may take actions at home to improve healing and minimize swelling. These might include using cold compresses, avoiding intense activity, and elevating your head while sleeping.

Your nose's appearance may vary gradually as it heals. Be patient and trust the process, since the ultimate results may take many months to emerge. If you have any questions or concerns throughout your recuperation, please do not hesitate to contact your healthcare team for advice and assistance.

Incorporating Rhinoplasty Results Into Your Daily Life

Once you've completely healed from rhinoplasty, integrating your new look into your everyday routine is a fascinating possibility. You may feel more secure and self-assured as you handle social and professional settings with your improved characteristics.

To maintain the benefits of your rhinoplasty, emphasize self-care and live a healthy lifestyle while you acclimate to your new face. This includes maintaining excellent skincare routines, preventing your face from UV damage, and avoiding activities that might jeopardize the integrity of your nose, such as smoking.

It's also vital to moderate your expectations and understand that rhinoplasty isn't a one-time cure, but rather a path of self-development. Accept the changes in your look as part of your continuing personal development and progress.

Remember that the choice to get rhinoplasty was made to boost your confidence and well-being. Celebrate your metamorphosis and embrace your newfound freedom to express yourself truthfully. With patience, positivism, and self-love, you may truly embrace your rhinoplasty results and enjoy life to the fullest.

CHAPTER 10

Alternatives To Rhinoplasty

Non-Surgical Solutions For Nasal Augmentation

Non-surgical solutions for nasal augmentation provide an alternative for those who want to change the look of their nose without having surgery. Dermal fillers are a typical non-surgical technique. These fillers, usually composed of hyaluronic acid, are injected into particular parts of the nose to reshape it, rectify asymmetry, or smooth out bumps and depressions. In comparison to surgery, the process is quite rapid and requires little downtime.

Another nonsurgical alternative is the use of neuromodulators such as Botox. While Botox is most recognized for its wrinkle-reducing properties, it may also be used to treat specific nasal issues.

For example, it may be injected into the muscles surrounding the nose to lessen the appearance of bunny lines or to gently raise the nose tip.

Non-surgical nose reshaping using threads has also gained favor in recent years. This treatment includes putting dissolvable threads into the nose to give structural support while also reshaping the nasal contour. While less intrusive than surgery, the results are just temporary and may need reapplication regularly to maintain the desired look.

Benefits And Drawbacks Of Non-Invasive Techniques

Non-invasive techniques for nasal augmentation have various advantages over conventional rhinoplasty. For starters, they often need less downtime, enabling people to return to their daily activities quickly after treatment. This makes them a suitable alternative for those who have hectic schedules or cannot take time off work for surgery.

Furthermore, non-invasive techniques are frequently less risky and have fewer possible problems than surgery. Because they do not need incisions or general anesthesia, the danger of scarring, infection, and other surgical complications is greatly decreased. Individuals who are afraid to have surgery may find this comforting.

However, non-invasive techniques do have limits that must be addressed. While they may generate considerable changes in nasal appearance, the outcomes are often transitory and may need continuous therapy. Furthermore, non-surgical methods may be ineffective for those who have significant nose abnormalities or structural difficulties that need surgical intervention to rectify.

Lifestyle Adjustments That Improve Nose Health And Attractiveness

In addition to medical treatments, several lifestyle adjustments may help improve nose health and appearance.

Maintaining general good health is critical, since issues such as smoking, poor diet, and dehydration may all have an impact on the nose's skin and cartilage.

A well-balanced diet high in vitamins and minerals may benefit skin health and encourage tissue regeneration, perhaps improving the look of the nose over time. Drinking enough water is also important for keeping the skin moisturized and avoiding dryness and flakiness.

Furthermore, healthy skincare practices may aid in the health and attractiveness of the nose. This involves frequently cleaning the skin to eliminate debris, oil, and pollutants, as well as using moisturizers and sunscreen to protect against sun and environmental damage.

Finally, avoiding habits that might harm the nose, such as frequent picking or rubbing, will help prevent injury and keep it in its natural form and symmetry.

Overall, making these lifestyle modifications may supplement medical treatments and contribute to a healthier, more appealing nasal look.

When Rhinoplasty May Not Be The Best Option

Rhinoplasty is a very efficient treatment for correcting nose abnormalities and improving facial harmony, but it may not be the best choice for everyone. In certain cases, other therapies or lifestyle adjustments may be more suited.

Individuals with excessive expectations or body dysmorphic disorder, for example, may not be suitable candidates for rhinoplasty since surgery alone will not treat underlying psychological difficulties. Similarly, people with certain medical illnesses or risk factors may not be good candidates for surgery because of the higher risk of complications.

Furthermore, some people may have minor nasal abnormalities that may not need surgical surgery. In certain circumstances, non-surgical treatments like dermal fillers or Botox may provide adequate results without the need for invasive surgery.

Finally, the choice to have rhinoplasty should be made in conjunction with a knowledgeable plastic surgeon who can evaluate the patient's specific requirements and objectives and offer the best treatment approach. A tailored strategy may be devised by taking into account elements such as the severity of the nasal issues, the individual's general health, and their aesthetic preferences.

Conclusion

To summarize, comprehending rhinoplasty is a multilayered journey through the complexities of nasal anatomy, surgical procedures, patient expectations, and post-operative care. This thorough book has shed light on the transformational power of rhinoplasty, including its artistic subtleties and medicinal relevance.

Rhinoplasty is fundamentally a cosmetic treatment that strikes a precise balance between form and function. Surgeons must manage the complicated interaction of nasal components to achieve both aesthetic harmony and proper breathing. They design the nose to suit the patient's distinct facial characteristics while resolving any functional problems.

Throughout this book, we have looked at the many reasons people choose rhinoplasty, including correcting congenital defects and improving face symmetry and self-confidence.

Each patient takes their unique set of objectives and concerns to the operating table, and it is the surgeon's responsibility to listen carefully and cooperate closely to accomplish the desired result.

Furthermore, we explored the numerous surgical methods and procedures used in rhinoplasty, emphasizing the need for customization and accuracy. Whether doing an open or closed treatment, the surgeon must use their knowledge to remodel the nasal structure with precision, providing natural-looking results while reducing the risk of problems.

However, the trip does not finish in the operation room. Post-operative care is critical to ensuring good recovery and long-term happiness. Patients must follow their surgeon's recommendations exactly, from controlling pain and swelling to protecting the nasal area from damage. Patients who follow these suggestions and attend follow-up consultations may nurture their newfound nasal aesthetics and confidently enjoy their improved look.

Ultimately, rhinoplasty is more than just a surgical procedure; it is a transforming experience that goes beyond physical changes. It can transform not only the nose but also one's self-image and quality of life. Understanding the complexities of rhinoplasty allows patients to begin on this road with confidence and educated decision-making, aided by their surgeon's knowledge and the support of their healthcare team.

Finally, the entire guide to understanding rhinoplasty is an invaluable resource for patients, doctors, and enthusiasts alike, encouraging a greater appreciation for the art and science of nasal surgery. As we continue to explore new frontiers in aesthetic medicine, let this information inspire people to achieve their aesthetic goals with confidence and elegance.

THE END